Diets to help
MULTIPLE SCLEROSIS

Provides a series of alternative diets, nutritious recipes and helpful advice regarding the management of this disease for individual cases.

Diets to help

MULTIPLE
SCLEROSIS

Helping to control symptoms naturally

RITA GREER

Thorsons
An Imprint of HarperCollins*Publishers*

Thorsons
An Imprint of HarperCollins*Publishers*
77–85 Fulham Palace Road,
Hammersmith, London W6 8JB

1160 Battery Street,
San Francisco, California 94111–1213

First published 1982
Second edition published 1990
This edition 1995
1 3 5 7 9 10 8 6 4 2

© Rita Greer 1982, 1995

Rita Greer asserts the moral right
to be identified as the author of this work

A catalogue record for this book
is available from the British Library

ISBN 0 7225 3239 3

Printed in Great Britain by
HarperCollinsManufacturing Glasgow

Contents

Introduction

We live in a time when there is a kind of desperation among researchers to crack the Multiple Sclerosis mystery. All kinds of theories abound, and there is a good deal of conflict of opinion as to the best way of coping with the disease, or whether indeed it is worth trying to do anything about it at all. The result of this is a kind of free-for-all of ideas, and it places both the patients and the experts in a curious dilemma. How should the MS patient be advised, and if the patient is advised should he or she take the advice offered?

What usually happens is that no advice whatsoever is offered regarding diet, or any other aspect of MS, and the patient consequently does nothing to change existing eating habits which may be appalling from a nutritional point of view. With over a hundred years of frustration behind it, regarding research into MS, the medical profession has tended to lose patience with both the disease and those with MS. It is not surprising then that some MS sufferers have in turn largely lost patience with their doctors.

Over the last two decades, several types of therapy have received media attention, regardless of whether or not they were effective for MS. They have ranged from injections of cobra venom to herculean exercise programmes and hyperbaric oxygen treatment. The more of these alternative treatments there are, the more the medical profession runs out of patience as in its world there is still nothing to offer. There are rumblings about gene therapy, and vast amounts of money have been spent on research, especially in the USA. There is a great deal of clutching at straws and, as more and more people are diagnosed every year, the desperation never really lets up.

This abysmal situation does at least leave one option open to those with MS – regarding diet they are free to captain their own ship. The first step is to decide what type of diet to follow, and trial, error and common sense will have to play a major part in the deciding.

Research has shown that people with MS fare better if they use diet and exercise as a way of trying to control the illness.

In this book I give very basic guidelines on the modern view of diets and MS. In the absence of a cure for the disease, sensible management and as much control over it as possible would seem to be the best course of action. Sitting about, passively waiting for the worst to happen is no course of action at all.

CHAPTER ONE

What Happens in MS?

MS (Multiple Sclerosis), or DS (Disseminated Sclerosis) as it is still sometimes called, is classed as a disease of the central nervous system. Nobody knows yet what causes it, although many theories have been put forward over the last hundred years or so.

Basically, the protective covering of the nerves becomes inflamed, or even scarred, causing disruption in the transmission of messages from the brain to one or many parts of the body. Bad scarring of the nerve covering (myelin sheath) can result in permanent disability. Some people experience a type of MS which slowly becomes worse; a kind of downward spiral of illness with more and more symptoms. Some patients experience pain, others do not. Some have had bouts of MS and then 'remissions' when they improve for a while. It is this coming and going of the disease which is one of its most puzzling aspects and one which makes it very difficult for researchers to make any progress.

As one or many parts of the body can be affected, and the severity and pattern of the MS can vary so much, the illness does not present itself in the same way in each person, i.e. there are no two cases the same.

A great deal of money has been spent on research into MS throughout the world, but so far very little has been learned. In the last few years the impatience of the mass of people with MS has shown itself in a new attitude of self-help, both in therapy and diet. This approach is largely frowned on by the medical profession, as it is with other degenerative diseases that cannot be cured by surgery or known drugs, but, interest in this new kind of attitude seems to be growing all the time.

IS DIET IMPORTANT?

That MS can be helped by diet alone is probably a foolish notion. Moderate lifestyle, adequate rest, suitable exercise and freedom from stress may all have an important part to play. But, there is no doubt that poor nutrition can actually cause illnesses such as rickets, anaemia, scurvy etc., and when a person already has an illness such as a heart disorder, colitis, MS etc. poor nutrition will make it even worse. If a healthy person needs a good diet to maintain health, a sick person needs a good diet to improve health and heal or control the illness that already exists.

Here is an example of the kind of daily menu that can only make matters worse for a sick person. Sadly, it is all too typical of the eating patterns of most people with MS, especially those who have to cope on their own. Convenience foods from the freezer, instant meals from tins and the like are the easiest to prepare and shop for, but they can represent a trap which may ensure continuing bad health.

AN EXAMPLE OF BAD EATING HABITS

Breakfast: Cereal with milk and sugar; a cup of tea with milk and sugar.

Elevenses: A cup of coffee with milk and sugar; biscuits or a chocolate bar.

Lunch: Tinned spaghetti in tomato sauce on white bread toast with butter; shop-bought cake or more biscuits; a cup of coffee with milk and sugar.

Tea: More biscuits; bread (white) with butter and jam.

Evening meal: Sausages or hamburger (fried in lard), tinned peas, instant mashed potato; tinned fruit in syrup with cream or ice cream.

Even the healthiest of people would be likely to succumb to some illness on such a diet, which usually does not vary from one day to the next. It has just about everything wrong with it. The diets that follow paint a different picture of nutrition altogether. They are designed to rectify our bad western eating habits.

One of the few discoveries about MS is that people with the illness have lower levels of linoleic acid in their red blood cells and body tissues than is considered normal. This can be taken into account when putting together a diet for someone with MS.

THE CONTROL OF SYMPTOMS

Very often MS patients experience constipation because of a change in their lifestyle, such as drastic reduction in physical activity, due mainly to the fatigue that comes with MS. This problem can often be alleviated by increasing the amount of bran in the diet, thus removing the need for laxatives which can deplete the body of much needed vitamins and minerals.

Some MS patients have found that certain other symptoms can be controlled by eliminating various foods from their diets. Shortness of breath, breathing difficulties and catarrh etc. sometimes respond to the removal of milk and milk products from the diet. In which case, substitute soya milk and use a multi-vitamin tablet that contains calcium.

Difficulty in adjusting to temperature changes, and the frequent running of above-normal body temperatures can sometimes be alleviated by cutting out cane and beet sugar. For this, fructose (fruit sugar) can be substituted. No supplement is necessary as sugar is only carbohydrate.

Fatigue that so often comes with MS can often be tackled by eating little and often, say five small meals a day instead of three large ones.

Worsening of symptoms and weakness can be helped by the avoidance of alcohol. Alcohol only makes existing symptoms more apparent, and it is especially bad for vertigo and balance generally. Substitute alcoholic drinks with imaginative fruit cocktails, herb teas and savoury drinks.

Stimulants such as strong tea and coffee can cause difficulties. Anything which stimulates a damaged nervous system including smoking should be avoided.

SUPPLEMENTS TO HELP YOU GENERALLY

Linoleic acid, only low values of which are found in the plasma, nerve tissues and red cells of people with MS, can be obtained together with gamma-linolenic acid from the oil of the evening primrose. This is available in capsule form and there are now many types on the market but in varying strengths and doses. Although some may look like bargains, the increased dose that needs to be taken really means that such capsules work out more expensive in the long run. There are reports of unscrupulous companies marketing blended vegetable oils and claiming them to be oil of evening primrose, but without the all-important gamma-linolenic acid, constituent. Other important acids of the alpha series can be obtained in some capsules together with linolenic acid and gamma-linolenic acid, important for the maintenance of healthy cell membranes of the brain and nervous system. The recommended daily dosage (backed by ethical research) is six capsules daily, each containing 500mg (or approximately 6ml) of oil of evening primrose. Each capsule will give linoleic acid (9:12 vitamin F) and gamma-linolenic acid (6:9:12, vitamin F) in what is thought to be the most effective amounts for the control of MS.

If you are going to take multi-vitamins then choose

one for general use. There is nothing to be gained by taking too many vitamins, and perhaps even less by taking the types of vitamin pills that should really be described as 'junk pills'. These are usually sugar coated and filled with chemicals and fillers such as lactose. Avoid capsules and tablets which do not make a full declaration of ingredients.

For specific use:

Vitamin E (200 iu) for healing and body efficiency.

Vitamin B_{12} (1000mcg). For those on a vegetarian diet (be sure to get the correct strength).

Vitamin C (500mg) for protection and general health.

Vitamin A and Vitamin D from halibut oil and cod liver oil for protection and general health. (*Do not exceed dose on pack.*) Alternatives for vegetarians are available at health-food shops.

A good and varied diet should mean there is no need for any supplements except perhaps the capsules which contain gamma-linolenic acid. Only when there are digestive troubles which prevent the eating of a healthy diet should supplements be used. Any categories of food that cannot be eaten comfortably should be balanced with an appropriate supplement; for example, if citrus fruit cannot be taken, then it is a good idea to take extra vitamin C.

WHICH DIET IS FOR YOU?

There is no single perfect diet for all cases of MS in all parts of the world. In this book I try to show the whole spectrum of diets for MS – those of the 'Establishment', of doctors with experience in treating MS, and also general health diets, exclusion diets and a very strict individually tailored diet.

For people with the benign form of MS I would suggest trying one of the two general health diets. People who have great faith in doctors could try one of the doctor's diets. Those who cannot tolerate wheat, gluten or milk will find the exclusion diets more likely to produce results.

Whichever diet you choose, give it a reasonable try and keep a record of how you feel week by week. If you choose a diet which is obviously not suited to your metabolism it would be unwise to pursue it. The object is to find a diet that will improve general health and comfortably manage the MS, reducing the severity of attacks that may occur.

A basic consideration is the availability of special foods. Living in a city is a complication when fresh farm produce is required daily. Being able to afford the special foods is yet another problem. Items such as game and expensive fish are way out of reach of most of us. Supplements, too, may be financially beyond our purses, however reasonably priced.

Yet another difficulty can be fitting a special diet, with its extra shopping and careful preparation, into an already overloaded household routine. The extra work involved may prove to be too much for the person who keeps house.

However, if a special diet can be started, just the psychological reaction in the patient of undertaking a positive step to combat the MS, instead of just waiting for the illness to worsen and doing nothing about it, is a bonus and well worth the effort. General health can improve greatly on a healthier diet than has been previously followed.

Fighting an incurable disease is hard work and the value of rest in the control of MS should not be underestimated. Smoking *must* be avoided, as well as smoky atmospheres. The rather miserable forecasts often made by doctors should not be taken too seriously. Most doctors base their experience of MS on the chronic hospitalized cases they have seen and not the larger section of the population who have MS, still mobile and with slight, if any, disabilities.

CHAPTER TWO

The Various Diets

Some readily available foods are of questionable value, and such items are not recommended as part of a good diet no matter what state of health the eater enjoys. Foods from the following lists should be restricted or even avoided altogether.

1 Fibre-depleted or low-fibre foods

Sugar and sugary foods such as sweets, chocolate, jams, tinned fruit, prepared pie fillings, instant puddings, ice cream, ready-made desserts, bakery items made with refined white flour, white bread.

2 Highly salted foods

Crisps, salted peanuts and snacks, smoked fish such as kippers, bacon, yeast extracts, salty spreads such as fish or meat pastes. Also avoid liberal use of salt in cooking and at the table. Some convenience foods can have

Diets to help MULTIPLE SCLEROSIS

unexpectedly high salt content – such as cornflakes and commercially made biscuits.

3 Complicated processed foods

Avoid foods which have had all kinds of chemicals added to improve colour, texture, flavour, appearance and shelf-life.

4 Cholesterol or saturated fat-rich foods

Cream, lard, dripping, cheeses, butter, fat meats such as pork and bacon, peanut butter, gold-top milk, commercial salad cream and mayonnaise, hard margarines, most nuts, sausages.

5 'Junk foods'

Those which are messed about so much they can hardly be described as nutritious. They come in tins and packets, in all shapes and sizes. They appear to be appetizing both in colour and texture, and they often taste nice, too!

DIET A
(General Health Diet for Meat and Fish Eaters)

All vegetables are suitable, but these are the most important in a diet for an MS patient:

12

Red Vegetables. Carrots, peppers, beetroot, tomatoes.

Green Vegetables. Kale, cabbage, broccoli/calabrese, spinach, peppers, beans (string, French, runner, stick), watercress.

Sprouted Seeds. Bean sprouts, cress etc.

Nuts and Seeds. Walnuts, almonds, sunflower seeds, sesame seeds.

Herbs and Spices. Fresh herbs such as parsley, sage, thyme, rosemary. Spices such as mixed spice, all-spice, coriander, cumin, nutmeg etc.

Bran. Cereal fibre of some kind is desirable – wheat or rice bran.

Bakery Items etc. Those made with wholewheat flour, wholewheat bread, (care must be taken to buy bread which is genuine wholewheat bread, not just white bread dyed brown), crispbreads such as *Ryvita*, wholewheat pastas.

Pulses. Peas, beans, lentils, split peas, broad beans.

Fruit. All fresh fruit except avocado pears.

Meat, Fish and Eggs. Fresh kinds of the less fatty types. Avoid sausages and hamburgers. Fresh farm eggs (up to three per week).

Oils and Fats. Sunflower oil, soya oil, soft margarines made with a high proportion of polyunsaturated fat.

Milk and Milk Products. Fresh milk (preferably butter-milk), low-fat dried milk, plain cottage cheese (without added cream), plain low-fat yogurt.

Sugar and Honey. Allowed in very small amounts.

Rice, Oats, Oatmeal.

Drinks. Weak tea, decaffeinated coffee, herb teas, fresh fruit and vegetable juices. If alcohol is tolerated and does not make symptoms worse, then stick to light wines (no spirits).

This list is a general one and does not take into account any special restrictions such as vegetarian food and gluten-free foods, or even foods which may cause discomfort, such as pulses. It probably represents the broadest kind of diet possible and the limits of a new kind of eating pattern that most people would wish to go to. More specialized diets follow later in the book.

If this general diet is followed there should be no need to supplement daily eating with any kind of vitamins and minerals. However, great care must be taken to eat substantial amounts of the second category – green vegetables – to maintain an adequate supply of folic acid. The general diet should be put together in the following proportions:

45 per cent fresh fruit and vegetables, including
    potatoes, herbs, spices and pulses.
20 per cent bakery items etc.
20 per cent meat, fish and eggs.
15 per cent fats, oils, dairy products, nuts and seeds.

Bear in mind that the following should be avoided or restricted:
    Fibre-depleted or low-fibre foods; highly salted and sugared foods; complicated processed foods; cholesterol or saturated fat-rich foods and 'junk foods'.
    Fresh foods must be eaten, not frozen or tinned, raw vegetables and fruit being preferable to cooked varieties.

Should this type of diet prove to be ineffectual, then a stricter one can be tried with added vitamins and minerals (see Recipe section for suitable recipes). See Chapter One for information on supplements.

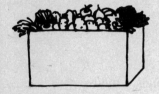 45% fresh fruit and vegetables

 20% bakery items

 20% meat, fish and eggs

 15% fats, oils, nuts and seeds

Proportions of Foods for Diet A

DIET B
(General Health Diet for Vegetarians)

Red Vegetables. Carrots, peppers, cabbage, beetroot, tomatoes,

Green Vegetables etc. Kale, cabbage, broccoli/calabrese, spinach, peppers, green beans, watercress, plus all other vegetables.

Sprouting Seeds. Bean sprouts, cress.

Nuts and Seeds. Walnuts, almonds, sunflower seeds, sesame seeds.

Herbs and Spices. All fresh herbs; all dried spices.

Bran. Wheat or rice bran.

Bakery Items etc. Wholewheat flour items, wholewheat bread; crispbreads such as *Ryvita;* wholewheat pastas.

Pulses etc. Peas, beans, lentils, split peas, broad beans.

Fruit. All fruit.

Eggs. Up to seven farm eggs, medium size, per week.

Oils and Fats. Sunflower oil, soya oil, olive oil, soft margarines, made with a high proportion of sunflower oil.

Milk and Milk products. Fresh skimmed milk or low-fat dried milk, plain low-fat yogurt, cottage cheese (without cream).

Sugar and Honey. Taken in very small amounts only.

Rice, Oats, Oatmeal.

Supplements – essential: Vitamin B_{12} (1000mcg) 1 per day.

The vegetarian diet should be put together in this way:

45 per cent fresh fruit and vegetables including potatoes.

20 per cent bakery items etc.
20 per cent pulses, eggs, dairy items.
15 per cent fats, oils, nuts and seeds.

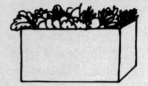

45% fresh fruit and
vegetables

20% bakery items

20% pulses, eggs and dairy
items

15% fats, oils, nuts and
seeds

Proportions of Foods for Diet B

Bear in mind that the following should be avoided or
restricted:

Fibre-depleted or low-fibre foods, highly salted foods, highly sugared foods, complicated processed foods, cholesterol or saturated fat-rich foods and 'junk foods'. (See previous diet for advice on alcohol.)

Fresh foods must be eaten, not frozen or tinned, raw vegetables and fruit being preferable to cooked types. Great care must be taken to eat substantial amounts of green vegetables to maintain an adequate supply of linoleic acid.

Should this type of diet prove to be ineffectual, then a stricter one can be tried with more vitamin and mineral supplements. See Chapter One for information on supplements.

DIET C
(Essential Fatty Acids Diet)

Some people only feel well when they can eat a good deal of meat and fish. The most basic of diets which will accommodate this is one which is just high in the essential fatty acids usually lacking in people with MS. These essential fatty acids have a better chance of getting to work if cholesterol and saturated fat-rich foods are largely avoided or cut down in the diet. Unfortunately, the two things have a habit of appearing together in foods so that while items like peanut butter may be rich in essential fatty acids, they are also loaded with saturated fat.

I give only a very basic outline of this diet here. Basically you would have to eat:

Lean meat, especially game;
organ meats, especially liver;
freshwater fish, marine fish and shellfish;
lots of fresh fruit and vegetables;
pulses and nuts;
sunflower seed oil, soya oil, sesame seed oil, olive oil
    and corn oil;
unrefined cereals and wholemeal bread;
pure honey, brown rice, raw sugar, eggs in moderation;
seasonings, herbs and spices.

DIET D

(The Bauer Diet from *A Manual on Multiple Sclerosis*
published by the International Federation of Multiple
Sclerosis)

This is a very general diet which should be arranged to
give 50 per cent carbohydrates, 30 per cent fats and 20
per cent protein with a daily calorific intake of 1,800
calories.

Basically, the diet should give sufficient but not too high
calorific intake; a limited amount of fats, high in polyunsaturates and providing a low cholesterol intake; a liberal
amount of animal and plant protein; a limited sugar
intake, but generous amounts of grains and potatoes;
liberal amounts of vegetables and fruit, preferably fresh.

Carbohydrates – bread (wholewheat and rye), rice, oats,
    oatmeal and other cereals, potatoes, (50 per cent).
    Limit cakes, sweets, sugar.

Fats – Sunflower oil, safflower oil, margarines high in polyunsaturates, (30 per cent). Eliminate as far as possible, butter, lard, fat bacon, fat meat.

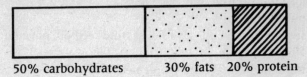

| 50% carbohydrates | 30% fats | 20% protein |

Proportions of Foods for Diet D

Proteins – soya, beans and peas (if tolerated); cottage cheese, low-fat yogurt; fish.

Meat – chicken, turkey, lean veal, beef, lamb, pork.

Avoid: fat bacon, sausages, kidney, brain. Grill or roast instead of frying. Restrict eggs.

Vegetables and Fruit – no restrictions.

Spices – no restrictions.

Drinks – fruit and vegetable juices (preferably fresh); buttermilk, skimmed milk; spring water, limited amounts of mineral water; coffee, tea; small quantities of light alcoholic drinks – beer, light wines – only if they do not impair co-ordination.

This is the 'establishment' view of diet for MS. Individuals such as Dr Evers and Professor Roy Swank have quite different ideas. Nevertheless, all these diets for MS patients have a few things in common; for example, a low cholesterol intake, a preference for oils high in polyunsaturates, the liberal use of fresh fruit and vegetables and the use of whole foods such as wholewheat bread as opposed to the more refined 'junk food' types. With so many schools of thought there are bound to be widely differing opinions. To take the broad view of the situation, the type of diet followed must take into account availability of food – both for type and quantity; the area of the world in which the patient lives and its traditional food habits; finance; a patient's limitations regarding the preparation of food, shopping etc. If the wrong diet is chosen for a particular person, the aggravation to that person and his or her family can cause a new kind of stress that totally negates any improvement that might take place in the patient's MS.

Undoubtedly, the most difficult diets to follow are the exclusion type where one or more basic items of a normal diet are taken out, such as wheat or milk.

DIET E
(Wheat Free Diet)

The basic items of this diet include: plenty of fresh vegetables; sunflower and sesame seeds, sprouting seeds such as cress and beanshoots; fresh or dried fruit (except avocado pears) walnuts, almonds; all kinds of spices and herbs; rice, ground rice, rice bran, maize flour, oats; dried peas and beans; grilled or roasted fresh meat with all visible fat trimmed off, game; poultry, (except duck and goose); white fish; skimmed milk or buttermilk, low-fat yogurt, cottage cheese, three fresh farm eggs per week; margarine (polyunsaturated), sunflower oil, soya oil; honey, Barbados sugar, black pepper, salt, thin wheat free soy sauces, wine or cider vinegar; fresh fruit juices, weak tea, decaffeinated coffee.

If alcohol is tolerated and gives no adverse effects

stick to light wines, in moderation, also sherry.

When wheat is left out of the diet, there may be a craving for bread. The following are expensive but are nutritious and wheat-free: *Trufree* Flours for bread etc. (Numbers 1 to 7). The diet can be followed without the special breads and flours but some people may find this a little boring, the main sources of starch being potatoes and rice. Some crispbreads on the market do not contain wheat, so look carefully at the labels before buying.

Regarding supplements; without bread there may be a fall in the consumption of yeast. This can be put right by taking brewer's yeast tablets and these will replace the lost B vitamins. A multi-vitamin can also be taken, along with Evening Primrose Oil containing gamma-linolenic acid, and if a reduction in protein intake occurs, soya protein tablets will help to rectify this.

A sudden weight loss may be experienced on this diet if previous levels of protein and starch are not maintained. Wheat bread in the normal diet accounts for about one sixth of an adult's daily protein intake and it is a high-carbohydrate energy food. A reduction in fibre intake may lead to constipation. This can be put right by using rice bran in baking or sprinkled over fruit.

DIET F
(Milk-free Diet)

The basic items of this diet include: all fresh vegetables; sunflower and sesame seeds; fresh fruit, walnuts, almonds; black pepper and spices, salt, raw sugar, honey; brown rice, wheat bran, wholemeal flour, wholewheat bread (baked at home); pulses such as dried peas and beans, lentils and split peas; fresh meat, game – meat must be lean and with fat trimmed off; poultry (except duck and goose); fish (fresh); up to three fresh farm eggs per week; sunflower oil, olive oil; fresh fruit juices, weak tea with fresh lemon, herb teas, decaffeinated coffee without milk. Alcoholic drinks should be limited to light wines, in moderation, if they can be tolerated.

There are a few margarines available that are milk-free but high in saturated fat – not advisable for people with MS. Instead of margarine or butter, sunflower or olive oil must be used. You may be able to find a commercially-baked bread that does not contain any milk products such as emulsifiers, but safest is home-baked wholewheat bread. Do not use margarine for greasing tins.

In the UK, vitamins A and D have to be added to margarines. It may be wise to supplement the diet with these especially during winter months. There are vitamin A, D and E tablets which do not contain lactose (a milk product) so read the labels carefully. Do not use commercial lemon juice in tea, however handy it might seem, as all kinds of chemicals are put in to preserve it.

Eat plenty of green vegetables and fresh fruit as in the 'General Health Diet' (Diet A).

As milk and milk products supply protein and calcium in the ordinary diet, a multi-vitamin that will make up the latter deficiency is a good idea. Protein can be made up with extra meat and fish and also soya milk.

DIET G
(Gluten-free Diet)

In the 1970s there was a good deal of publicity for this type of diet, normally used to control coeliac disease, because claims were made that it was the cure for MS. Interest in the theory first began as far back as the 1950s when an Australian researcher linked the high incidence of MS in areas of high cereal production with consumption of cereals in the diet. The cause was taken up by the late Roger McDougall who claimed his MS had benefitted greatly from it. In spite of a great deal of scorn from the medical profession, many MS patients seized on this diet as the answer to their predicament, without any hard evidence of cures having taken place.

Gluten is found in wheat, rye, barley and oats – only in these four grains, not in any other kind of basic food. The problem is that they are used in a great many other processed foods as binders, thickeners, coatings etc. Avoiding them all is not easy but it does stop the patient eating a great many junk foods. All meat, fish, fruit, vegetables, rice and milk are gluten-free so there is a wide range of basic food on which to structure the diet. Unfortunately, most of the commercially made gluten-free foods such as bread and biscuits are labelled 'gluten free' when in fact they are not gluten-free at all, so gluten-free baking is best done at home. This may make an extra burden on the MS patient or his/her carer, so a gluten-free diet should not be undertaken lightly. Unless a patient shows intolerance to gluten (an allergy), or experiences discomfort after food containing gluten is eaten, there would seem to be little point in a gluten-free diet. The cereals which don't contain gluten are principally rice and maize. If you want to follow this diet use the wheat-free diet as a basis (Diet E), but omit oats, and crispbreads. All *Trufree* flours are 100 per cent gluten-free, (numbers 1 to 7), and so are suitable. However, they are expensive and the diet can be maintained without them. Use the same supplements as recommended for the wheat-free diet; also follow the advice regarding sudden weight loss.

This diet will stop you eating ordinary sugary and starchy bakery items and many junk foods.

For help with a gluten-free diet, see the Appendix at the back of the book.

DIET H
(The Greer Diet)

This diet gained popularity in the 1970s when there was a great deal of publicity for it worldwide. It has subsequently been used to treat other degenerative illnesses as well as MS. As the media spread the word in what was not always an accurate way, so the myth of the diet grew. The man for whom the diet was designed spent years denying he had been cured of MS by using the diet. To get the diet in perspective, it is as well to look at the background to the myth and the diet itself.

Alan Greer was diagnosed as having severe MS in 1970. He was written off by doctors and given no more than 18 months to live. Instead of dying he made an amazing recovery and got back to something like a normal life. He made several changes to his life: he retired from work, he exercised within his capabilities daily and he changed his diet completely because some foods made him feel worse. By 1977 he had not only survived but improved so much that people began to question the diagnosis. A newspaper paid for him to be diagnosed again by the same specialist at a London hospital. Against all hopes, again he said it was MS.

By now the idea of exercise, some kind of diet and a more positive attitude had taken hold, and whereas in the past patients were just sent home from diagnosis in hospital and written off, a new attitude emerged. The charity Association for Research into MS was set up and there were diet trials and therapy groups.

In the early 1980s, Alan Greer's symptoms began to change, but it took until 1992 for a brain tumour to be diagnosed. He underwent major surgery for the partial removal of the tumour when it was discovered that there were no signs of MS. The surgeon thought the tumour had been growing for about 16 years but this did not explain the previous 20 or so years of MS symptoms.

As well as changing his diet drastically, Alan Greer took dietary supplements. He was the first person to take oil of evening primrose in the early 1970s, long before it was on the market. Now it is a commodity and sold in every chemist. He also took vitamin B_{12}. It has now been proven that people with MS have low levels of this vitamin. A multivitamin with a broad range of vitamins and minerals completed the dietary supplements. It is important to understand how the supplements balanced up the very unusual diet which cut out the three major allergens in the UK – wheat, milk and eggs. It also excluded cane and beet sugar, except for a minute quantity, and meat in all forms. Many people have found this extraordinary diet, which was tailored by trial and error for one man, to be of benefit. However, it obviously would not suit everyone.

The diet is included in this book because it forms part of the background to using diet to try and control MS.

Fats. Sunflower oil for salad oil, soya oil and corn oil; Flora margarine – 2 oz (50g) per day.

Starch/Cereals/Pulses. Maize meal, rice, ground rice; lentils, split peas; potatoes; Trufree Crispbran; rice bran.

Protein. Cod, haddock, plaice; natural flavour Protoveg (soya meat); walnuts, almonds; *Heinz* baked beans (about ½ medium-sized tin per day); soya flour and *Tamari* soy sauces (wheat/gluten free).

Fruit. All fresh fruit except avocado pears, all dried fruit except candied peel and dates rolled in sugar.

Sugar. Fructose (fruit sugar).

Drinks. Lemon tea with fresh lemon, fresh or tinned fruit juices without sugar, home-made soups, fresh vegetable juices, occasionally a small glass of white wine or sherry.

Vegetables. All fresh vegetables, raw or lightly cooked, lots of greens every day.

Seasoning and Spices. Salt, pepper (black), cinnamon, mixed spice etc; wine or cider vinegar.

Treats. Sugar-free jams (from health-food shops).

Essential Diet Supplements. Evening primrose oil (500mg);

Cantamac Tablets and *Cemac* Vitamin B_{12} (1000mcg).

Trufree 100 per cent wheat-free flours may also be used to add variety. For best results, all food must be eaten fresh, rather than tinned or frozen.

DIET I
(The Evers Diet)

Here is an example of a diet for MS designed by a doctor (Dr Paul Evers) who has a clinic in Germany and has had many years of experience in treating MS patients. An individual approach, it differs in many ways from other diets in this book.

There are three basic rules.

1 Eat vegetable foods instead of animal fats.
2 Of the fats eaten, more than half should be high in polyunsaturated fatty acids.
3 Avoid a high calorie intake.

Foods especially recommended are:

Fresh and dried fruits, eaten raw;
whole grains, fresh nuts, raw vegetables, leaf and root;
wholewheat bread, natural honey, farm eggs (fresh and free-range), milk and milk products fresh from the farm, cheeses, all natural types;
farm butter, sunflower oil, safflower oil, wheat germ oil, maize germ oil.

If the patient improves on this selection of foods he or she is then allowed:

Smoked meat, fresh salmon, raw ham, raw lean meat, freshwater fish, game and poultry, all herbs.

Dr Evers recommends these daily amounts of food:

Germinated grain – 2–4 oz (50-100g)
Wholewheat bread – up to 6 slices
Rolled oats – 3 oz (75g)
Fruit and vegetables – 1lb (450g)
Milk (with meals) – about 2 pints (1 litre)
Butter – about 1 oz (25g)
Honey – as desired
Linseed, sunflower seed and fresh nuts – about 4 oz (120g)
One egg

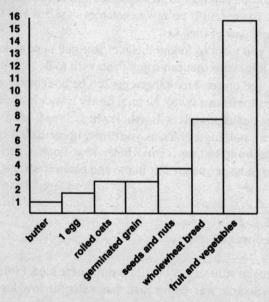

Daily amounts of foods for Diet I in 1 oz units

On very special occasions a glass of wine or beer.

Avoid junk foods: White sugar products, sweets, chocolate; white flour products, white bread, cakes, biscuits, pastries; preserves and tinned fruits, highly spiced foods, mustard, vinegar, saccharin, coffee.

Special containers for germinating seeds can be bought at good Health Food Stores.

Bear in mind that this diet was designed in Germany where the types of food which make up the national diet are different from those in the UK.

The food Dr Evers recommends is plain fare and should be eaten in as fresh and natural a state as possible. The accent is on raw vegetables so salads will form a basic part of this diet.

If you want to follow this diet you will need to know of a local farm that can supply you with milk, milk products and butter. Free-range eggs can be bought at health shops (or from a farm). Natural honey is widely available from health shops as is wholewheat bread, although, there's nothing as nice as your own home-baked bread made from 100 per cent wholewheat flour. Grain will need to be germinated at home and eaten fresh.

DIET J
(The Swank Diet)

Trying to control MS by diet is not a new idea. Professor Roy Swank was doing just that with his low-fat diet many years ago in Canada, and he is still doing so today. Bear in mind that this is a diet that was designed before oil of evening primrose was available, and before the arrival of soft margarines high in polyunsaturates.

Oils, to be taken: up to 4 teaspoonsful per day for inactive people, up to 8 teaspoonsful per day for active people and up to 10 teaspoonsful per day for very active people.

Nut and Seed Oils: Sunflower, safflower, soya, peanut, corn, olive, linseed.
Fish Oils. Cod liver, tuna, salmon, sardine, herring, mackerel.

Eat these foods in moderation (up to 3 units per day):

Each of these items = 1 unit for every 3 oz (75g). Chicken, beef, veal or pig's liver, calf or beef heart, veal, lamb or pig's kidney, leg of lamb, calf tongue, venison.
Each of these items = 1 unit for every 2 oz (50g). Lean beef, dark chicken and turkey meat without skin, chicken and turkey hearts, lamb's heart, lean ham, beef kidney, rib loin or shoulder of lamb, pheasant (without skin), lean pork, rabbit, beef tongue, veal.
Each of these items = 1 unit for every 1 oz (25g). Bacon, duck.

Avoid the following foods:
Dairy Produce. Whole milk, cream, butter, sour cream, ice cream, any kind of cheese and imitation dairy products.

Fats and Oils. Hard margarines, lard, chocolate, cocoa butter, coconut, coconut and palm oils.

Packet Foods. Cake mixes, biscuit and pastry mixes, potato crisps and snacks.

Bakery Items. Shop-bought pies, cakes, pastries, doughnuts, biscuits.

Tinned Foods. Any which contain cream, meat or dairy foods.

Meat and Poultry. Luncheon meats, salami, frankfurters, sausages, tinned meat products.

Supplements to take:
Vitamin E
1 teaspoonful of cod liver oil or 6-8 capsules per day
Multi-vitamin tablets or capsules
(Follow doses on packs)

Eat as much as you like of these foods:
Egg white, white fish, shellfish, poultry (breast with skin removed);

skimmed milk, buttermilk and low-fat milk (dried), low fat cottage cheese (rinsed under the tap), low-fat yogurt;

wholewheat bread, matzos, whole grain cereals, rice, wholewheat pasta, corn meal;

all fresh fruit and vegetables (steamed or raw), frozen or canned vegetables without butter;

jam, marmalade, honey, sugar, molasses, treacle, maple syrup, jelly.

CHAPTER THREE

Recipes

Healthy Chips

Here is a way of cooking chips that is not dangerous (no pan of hot oil), low in fat (only 1%) and easy. Cut up peeled, old potatoes into chips in the usual way. Spread out in a baking tin and, for every medium-sized potato, spoon in 1 teaspoonful of olive oil. Turn the chips over by hand to coat with the oil, wipe your hands on kitchen paper and put the chips into the oven on the top shelf at 450°F/230°C (Gas Mark 8).

Leave to cook for about 25 minutes, until crisp and golden, then serve right away.

• Suitable for all diets in this book.

Green vegetables are of prime importance in diets for MS.

How to Cook Spinach

Fill the kitchen sink with cold water and put in the spinach leaves. Thoroughly wash them and empty the

Diets to help MULTIPLE SCLEROSIS

sink. Rinse each leaf under the cold tap and put aside.
Now tear the leaves from the stems (discarding the
stems). Any tender looking stalks can be left on young
leaves. Choose a large saucepan, and cram it with the
leaves as they will shrink to a handful during cooking.
Don't put any water in the saucepan, but put over a low
heat and poke the leaves down as they cook. Gradually
bring to the boil in their own juice, adding a little salt to
encourage this. Put the lid on and cook for about 10
minutes or until tender. Strain in a colander while you
chop the cooked spinach with a sharp knife. This helps
to drain it and also make the cooked spinach more
manageable on the plate! If allowed, serve with a knob
of polyunsaturated margarine on a hot plate.

The strainings can be saved and used in gravy or in
soup and need not be washed, although ideally there
should be very little liquid to strain.

- Suitable for all diets in this book.

How to Cook Greens

Greens are a lifeline to any patient with MS and should
be eaten every day without fail. Overcooking must be
avoided at all costs and so must the old fashioned prac-
tice of boiling them in 'gallons' of water. The most effective way of cooking greens is to have just enough water
in the saucepan to stop them sticking or burning and to
make enough steam to cook them lightly.

Prepare the greens – choose whatever is in season
from dark green cabbage, spring greens, sprout tops,
kale and curly kale, broccoli or calabrese – washing

thoroughly in cold water. Cut or pull leaves away from main stalks and cut out and discard anything which does not look fresh or tender. While you are doing this you can be boiling ¼ inch water, with a few pinches of salt, in a large saucepan. Put in the prepared leaves etc. a few pieces at a time, poking them down with a wooden spoon until they have all been put in. This should keep the water boiling. Put the lid firmly on the saucepan and turn the heat to allow the greens to cook gently for about 7 to 10 minutes. Watch the saucepan does not go dry. If it does, add a little more water. Ideally you should have lightly cooked greens with little or no water to strain off. Put into a colander and snip with kitchen scissors for easy eating. Serve hot, immediately.

It is such a pity that so many people are put off eating greens because at an early age they have had mushy, soggy and slimy substances plonked on their plates. If you cook them in the way suggested you will find them full of flavour and an entirely different kind of proposition.

• Suitable for all diets in this book.

How to Cook Beans

Runner beans. Wash and trim off the tops, tails and strings using a small sharp kitchen knife. If you come across any which are obviously too tough, discard them. Slice through at an angle into equally-sized pieces. Put into boiling salted water, enough to come half way up the level of the beans. Cook with the lid on for 10 to 15 minutes for young beans and 20 to 25 minutes for end-of-season beans. Strain and serve right away.

French beans or green beans: Wash and just cut off the tops and tails. Cut into 2 inch long pieces. Cook as for runner beans but they will need only 7 to 10 minutes.

String beans: Prepare and cook as for French beans.

Beans from the freezer are not as good as fresh ones, either for nourishment or taste. Any cooked beans left over can be used as a salad. Sprinkle with a little finely chopped onion and pour over a little oil and vinegar dressing.

• Suitable for all diets in this book.

How to Cook Peas

Fresh peas: So much better than tinned or frozen ones which are all too often dyed to make them green. Shell the peas into a colander. Have ready boiling about ¼ inch lightly salted water. Put in the peas and cook with the lid on for about 10 minutes for young peas and up to 10 minutes longer for older peas. Strain and serve immediately.

Any cooked peas left over can be served in a salad or with finely chopped onion sprinkled over them.

• Suitable for all diets in this book.

Dried (Split) Peas: The most digestible form in which to serve these is probably in a soup.

Split Pea Soup

½ lb (225g) split peas
1 large onion, peeled and sliced
1 oz (25g) margarine (polyunsaturated)
1 pint (550ml) water
1 tablespoonful of thin soy sauce – or 2 teaspoonsful
   Marmite
½ lb (225g) carrots, trimmed, scrubbed and sliced
salt and freshly ground black pepper to taste.

Put the split peas into a fine mesh sieve and wash
thoroughly under the cold tap. Put into a large bowl
with about 1½ to 2 pints water. Leave to swell for about
12 hours.

Fry the onion in the margarine for about 4 minutes.
Pour in the pint of water and the soy sauce. Strain the
soaked split peas and add to the saucepan with the
carrots and a little salt. Bring to the boil and simmer
gently, with the lid on, for about 1 to 1¼ hours. Give it
a stir from time to time and if you find the soup going
too thick add a little more water. Season to taste.

For the most easily digested split pea soup, allow to
cool and then liquidize in a blender. This makes a very
filling soup.

• Suitable for all diets in this book.

Lentil Soup

Like split pea soup, lentil soup also makes use of a
pulse. Pulses are a much neglected part of our diet.

They are useful in removing toxins from the body and are high in fibre too.

5 oz (150g) lentils
2 medium-sized onions,
1 medium-sized potato, peeled and thinly sliced
2 tablespoonsful of sunflower or soya oil
1 pint (550ml) water
1 tablespoonful of soy sauce*
salt and freshly ground black pepper.

Wash the lentils in a wire sieve. Soak overnight in a large bowl with about 1 pint water. Fry the onion in the oil using a large saucepan. Add the soy sauce, strained lentils, the pint of water plus a little salt. Bring to the boil and simmer for about 40 minutes. Remove from heat, allow to cool and liquidize for a smooth and creamy soup. Reheat to serve.

• Suitable for all diets in this book if a gluten/wheat free soy sauce is used. Alternatively, use 2 teaspoonsful Marmite.

Parsley Soup

1 small onion, peeled and thinly sliced
1 heaped teaspoonful of polyunsaturated margarine or
   2 teaspoonsful of sunflower oil
2 oz (50g) fresh parsley, chopped and stems
   removed
2 medium-sized potatoes, peeled and sliced thinly
3 teaspoonsful of soy sauce or 1½ teaspoonsful of
Marmite

1 pint (550ml) skimmed milk or, if not allowed, use
  water
sea salt and freshly ground black pepper.

Fry the onion in the margarine or oil for 3 or 4 minutes.
Add the potato and parsley. Stir for a minute or two and
then add the milk or water. Bring to the boil and simmer
with the lid on for about half an hour. Remove from the
heat and allow to cool for a few minutes. Liquidize and
return to the saucepan. If it turns out too thick, add a
little water. Taste and season. Allow to cool and then
put into the fridge to chill for an hour. Serve cold.

   This soup can also be served hot after liquidizing and
is a good recipe for summer when greens are scarce.

   • Suitable for all diets in this book if gluten/wheat
free soy sauce is used.

Watercress Soup

1 medium-sized onion, peeled and thinly sliced
1 oz (25g) margarine if allowed, or 3 teaspoonsful of
  sunflower oil
1 bunch watercress including stems, washed thoroughly
  (discard any yellowing leaves), and coarsely
  chopped
¾ pint (415ml) water
2 teaspoonsful of soy sauce or 1 teaspoonful Marmite.

Fry the onion in the margarine or oil until transparent
but do not let it brown. Put in the watercress and about
half the water. Pour into the liquidizer and blend. Add

the rest of the water and the soy sauce. Bring to the boil and simmer for 10 minutes. Serve hot, or, allow to cool and chill in the fridge to serve cold. Season with salt just before serving, hot or cold.

• Suitable for all diets in this book.

BAKING YOUR OWN BREAD

No matter what advertisers say about commercially baked bread, there is nothing as nice or as good as home-baked bread. Here is a selection of recipes for ordinary and special breads. You will find less salt in these recipes than is normally used.

Wholewheat Bread

2 lb (900g) 100 per cent wholewheat flour
½ level teaspoonful of salt
½ oz (15g) active dried yeast
lukewarm water
1 heaped teaspoonful of Barbados sugar or fructose
   (whichever you are allowed).

First warm the bowl, either in the oven or in hot water, drying it thoroughly if you use the latter method. Put about ½ a cupful of warm water into a jug and sprinkle in the dried yeast and the sugar. Leave to let the yeast work. It should start to froth and go into bubbles. Put the flour into the warmed bowl and make a well in the centre. Stir the yeast mixture and when it has 'worked' pour into the well. Sprinkle the salt over the flour. Add more warm water (about a pint) and mix with a wooden spoon. You should have a fairly wet, soft mixture. (If you have put in too much water don't panic because you can add more flour later.) Cover the bowl with a clean tea cloth and leave in a warm place for the dough to rise to double its size. This can be in the airing cupboard, over the stove, over a radiator or a warm place in the sun – whatever is available.

When the dough has risen, dip you hands in flour and mix again, adding more flour. (You will find the dough will collapse back to its original size.) Then knead it for 3 or 4 minutes until you have a tough, pliable dough, all the time using more flour. Divide into 2 equal amounts and shape so you can drop it into 2 small, oiled tins. (Use sunflower oil.) Cover the tins with the clean cloth and leave to rise again in a warm place. This time let the dough rise by one half as much and bake in a preheated oven, above the middle shelf, 400°F/200°C (Gas Mark 6) for about 30 to 35 minutes. When they are cooked the loaves will sound hollow if you tap the tops. Turn out of the tins as soon as they come out of the oven and cool the loaves on a wire rack.

You will find this bread keeps longer than commercially produced bread without losing its wonderful flavour. If you find it goes stale too quickly, add a tablespoonful of sunflower oil to the flour and rub in before you start. Some people get best results by warming the flour in the bowl before they start.

If you feel you cannot get to grips with making your own bread on your own, find someone who makes their own and ask if they would be kind enough to show you how it is done. If using instant/easy blend yeast, add it dry to the flour. Up to 2 oz (50g) wheat-germ can be added to the flour.

• Suitable for all diets in this book except E, G and H.

Soda Bread (wholewheat)

About 1 lb (450g) wholewheat flour
1 level teaspoonful salt
1½ level teaspoonsful of bicarbonate of soda
½ pint (275ml) skimmed milk or reconstituted dried low-
    fat milk (if allowed), warm water.

The flour, salt and bicarbonate of soda must be thoroughly mixed. The best way to do this is to sieve it into a bowl, twice. Work in the milk as quickly as you can to make a soft dough. Add warm water if it is too stiff. (Hot water will make the soda over-react). Shape the dough into a flattish round and place on a floured baking sheet. Cut a cross on the top using a knife dipped in flour. Put straight into a pre-heated oven at 450°F/230°C (Gas Mark 8). Bake for about half an hour. Cool on a wire rack.

• Suitable for all diets in this book except E, G and H.

Gluten-free and Wheat-free Bread

Just under ½ pint (275ml) warm water
2 slightly heaped teaspoonsful of dried yeast granules
1 oz (25g) soya flour

4½ oz (115g) potato flour
3 oz (75g) maize flour
¾ oz (20g) yellow split pea flour or ground rice
¾ oz (20g) ground almonds
2 level teaspoonsful of dried pectin (liquid types are no
   good for this)
1 level teaspoonful of fructose or Barbados sugar,
   whichever is permitted
3 pinches salt
3 teaspoonsful of sunflower oil

Pre-heat oven at 350°F/180°C (Gas Mark 4). Sprinkle
the yeast into the warm water and leave for 3 or 4 minutes to soften. Put all other ingredients into a mixing
bowl and mix well, or, put through a sieve twice and
then into the bowl. Stir the yeast and water and pour
on to the blended four. Beat with a wooden spoon until
you have a thick batter.

Grease a medium-sized loaf tin (7¼ x 3½ x 2¼ inches,
185 x 90 x 50mm) with sunflower oil and flour, using
potato or maize flour. Put the mixture into this and
bake for 1 hour on the top shelf of the oven until light
brown and crusty. Turn out on to a wire rack to cool.
Use as ordinary bread. Store in a plastic bag, sealed. Do
not cut loaf until it is cold.

 • Suitable for diets E, G and H.

Gluten-free Fruit Tart

This recipe is also wheat-free

Pastry
2 oz (50g) polyunsaturated margarine
4 oz (100g) ground rice
3 oz (75g) finely grated eating apple (leave the skin on)

Filling
any kind of sweetened, stewed fruit using permitted sugar.

Use a form to blend the pastry ingredients then knead with the hands to form one ball. Grease an oven-proof pie plate and put the dough in the centre. Flatten with the palm and fingers until it has spread evenly over the bottom. Use the fingers to raise an edge all the way round. Bake in a pre-heated hot oven at 425°F/220°C (Gas Mark 7) for about 20 minutes until golden. Spread with hot stewed fruit and serve. This can also be eaten cold. If the stewed fruit turns out too thin then thicken with gluten-free maize flour before you finish cooking it.

• Suitable for diets E, G and H.

Fruit-on-Bread Pudding

This is a good way of using up special bread which would otherwise be wasted. Fry, on both sides, slices of thickly cut bread. Put on to a hot plate and top with stewed fruit sweetened with permitted sugar. This sounds a very simple dish but it is really delicious and very quick to make.

Best kinds of fruit are: blackberry and apple, gooseberries, damsons and plums, cherries. Use sunflower oil
for frying.

• Suitable for all diets in this book, but for diets A, B,
C, D, F, I and J use wholewheat bread and for diets E, G
and H use gluten-free bread.

All the experts agree on the value of salads for
people with MS. The dressings to moisten the salads
give an opportunity to use sunflower or soya oil which
are also important in diets for MS patients.

Oil and Vinegar Dressing

½ level teaspoonful of salt
a good sprinkling of black pepper, if allowed
1 tablespoonful of wine or cider vinegar
3 tablespoonsful of sunflower oil

Put all ingredients into a screw-top jar and shake vigorously to combine them. Store in the fridge and use as
required after shaking well.

• Suitable for all diets in this book.

Lemon Dressing

1 tablespoonful of fresh lemon juice
3 tablespoonsful of oil – sunflower or soya
½ teaspoonful of fructose or 1 teaspoonful of Barbados
    sugar, if allowed
salt and pepper to taste

Put all ingredients into a screw-top jar and blend well by shaking vigorously. Store in the fridge and use as required. Shake well before using.

• Suitable for all diets in this book.

Red Salad

Combine a selection of the following and dress with either of the two dressings suggested:

Chopped tomatoes
shredded red cabbage
finely chopped red peppers
grated carrot

For variation you might like to add finely grated apple or raisins. Beetroot, grated raw can also be added. This had a distinct earthy taste and makes a very moist salad.

• Suitable for all diets in this book.

Green Salad

Combine a selection of salad greens:

Cos lettuce
tender kale leaves
young leaves of spinach
green peppers chopped finely
watercress
Use either oil and vinegar dressing or lemon dressing.
Raw sprouts or cabbage can also be used.

• Suitable for all diets in this book.

Mixed Root Salads
(suitable for all diets in this book).

Finely grate and combine the following or any combination, according to season and availability:

carrot
parsnip
turnip
swede
courgettes
beetroot (raw)

Add a few chopped dates or sultanas and dress with either olive oil and vinegar dressing or lemon dressing.

Winter Salad

Combine a selection of the following and use either of the two dressings suggested:

Finely shredded red cabbage
Little Gem lettuce leaves
chopped fennel
tomato
celery or red pepper
grated carrot

• Suitable for all diets in this book.

Salad with Almonds

Make a mixture of three kinds of lettuce. Dress with the Oil and Vinegar Dressing and a sprinkle of sugar, salt and freshly ground black pepper. Scatter toasted almonds over the top and serve. Makes a good starter.

• Suitable for all diets in this book.

Unusual salad items can bring variety of taste and texture. Try raw chopped cauliflower florets, beanshoots, mushrooms, chopped walnuts or almonds.

Fruit can often be added to salads to give a sweeter taste – try grated apple, segments of orange or grapefruit, de-seeded grapes, slices of fresh peach or chopped dried prunes (stones removed) and dried apricots.

For salads with a bit of a crunch try adding cress, sunflower and sesame seeds as well as permitted nuts.

Fish Casserole

People who have to eat fish on special diets often get fed up with just fried or steamed dishes. Fish baked in a casserole is much more interesting and saves a lot of greasy washing up too.

1 medium-sized leek
½ green pepper de-seeded
1 oz (25g) permitted margarine or 1 tablespoonful of
    sunflower oil
¼ pint (140ml) water + 2 tablespoonsful of tomato
    purée, mixed well

2 medium-sized tomatoes
salt and pepper
about ½ lb (225g) haddock or cod fillet (fresh)
1 tablespoonful of lemon juice
2 heaped teaspoonsful of finely chopped fresh parsley.

Pre-heat oven to 350°F/180°C (Gas Mark 4) and put in
an oven-proof casserole to warm. Prepare the leeks and
cut into smallish pieces with the green pepper. Melt the
margarine (or heat the oil) in a medium-sized saucepan
and stir-fry for 7 to 8 minutes until the leek and green
pepper are tender, adding the tomato mixture after the
first 4 minutes. Remove from heat and put in the tomatoes, cut into 4 pieces. Season and put into the
warmed casserole. Cut the fish into two portions and
place on top. Pour the lemon juice over the fish.
Sprinkle all over with the chopped parsley and bake in
the oven with the lid on for 15 minutes. If the fillet is a
thick one, allow an extra 5 minutes.
Serve with hot brown rice or potatoes. Serves two.
• Suitable for all diets in this book.

Stir-fry Mixed Vegetables

Prepare vegetables – onion, carrot, parsnip or swede,
cabbage leaves, potato, tomato etc. as in season (any
vegetables will do, but you must start with an onion).

Slice the prepared vegetables thinly. Into a large frying pan with sloping sides, pour a little oil – about 2
tablespoonsful of sunflower or soya oil – and add the
sliced onion. Cook for 2 or 3 minutes until soft, then

add the rest of the vegetables in order of hardness, root vegetables first and soft things like cucumber and tomatoes last. Keep stirring the raw vegetables into the middle of the pan, turning them over gently. If it gets a little dry and they begin to stick, then add a little water. All the natural juices of the vegetables will blend. They should be cooked only very lightly, enough to make them tender enough to eat. Cooking takes only a few minutes. To make gravy add 2 to 3 teaspoons thin soy sauce to the juices. Serve hot immediately.

This method of cooking ensures maximum flavour and nutrition. Fresh vegetables in season must be used, not frozen or tinned.

• Suitable for all diets in this book if gluten/wheat free soy sauce is used.

Sweet and Sour Sauce

This is a useful, tasty sauce to serve on plain baked fish or as part of a Chinese-style meal with rice and stir-fry vegetables with fish. Makes 4 generous servings.

1 tablespoonful sunflower oil
1 medium onion, finely chopped
¼ green pepper, chopped
2 oz (50g) mushrooms, chopped
1 heaped tablespoonful fructose
2 tablespoonsful wine vinegar
1 level tablespoonful ground rice
1½ tablespoonsful tomato purée
½ pint (300ml) water

juice of 1 orange
1½ tablespoonsful soy sauce (wheat/gluten free if
   necessary)
3 pinches salt

Heat the oil in a medium-sized pan and add the onion.
Fry gently while you stir for 2 minutes. Add the green
pepper and mushrooms and stir-fry for another minute.
Remove from the heat. Mix the remaining ingredients
in a basin and poor into the pan. Heat and stir while it
thickens into a rich, red sauce.
• Suitable for all diets in this book.

Wholewheat Pasta

Once you have tried home-made pasta you will know
just how good pasta can be. It bears very little relation
to the white and tasteless varieties sold so widely.
   This recipe makes nearly ½lb (225g). It is nicest
cooked and eaten straightaway, but can be kept
uncooked in the fridge in a polythene bag for 1 or 2
days until required.

3 oz (75g) wholewheat flour
1 small egg
1-1½ tablespoonsful of sunflower or olive oil
3 pinches salt
a little water

Put the flour into a large mixing bowl. Sprinkle with
the salt. Make a well in the centre and pour in the egg,

lightly beaten with the oil. Use a fork to start mixing it all together. Add a little water, 1 spoonful at a time to bring together all the loose flour. Knead by hand for a few minutes on a floured surface until the dough becomes smooth and begins to look shiny. Cover with a clean teacloth and leave for about 10 to 15 minutes. Use plenty of flour to roll out the dough as thinly as you can. Cover the surface with a dusting of flour and roll up in a long sausage shape. Cut into thin slices to make long strips of pasta. These can be unrolled for cooking. (If you press the dough too hard while you cut it up it will all stick together so use a very sharp knife).

To cook: Bring a large pan of slightly salted water to the boil. Drop in the pasta and bring back to the boil. Cook steadily for about 6 minutes until softened but still on the firm side. You may need to give it a stir to separate the pieces. Strain in a colander. Put back into the saucepan and toss in a teaspoonful or two of sunflower oil. Sprinkle with black pepper and serve immediately. If not allowed cheese on your diet then sprinkle with Almond cheese (see next recipe).

• Suitable for diets A, B, C, D, F, I, J.

Almond Cheese

1 teaspoonful of sunflower oil
½ clove garlic, peeled,
3 pinches of salt
1 oz (25g) ground almonds
about 8 drops of lemon juice

Put the oil and salt into a small basin. Rub the cut part of the garlic clove around the basin, spreading the oil and salt. Discard the garlic. Put in the ground almonds and mix with a fork to absorb the oil. Add the lemon juice and mix in lightly. Leave for 12 hours to dry out. Use instead of Parmesan cheese for sprinkling over pasta.

• Suitable for all diets in this book.

Almond Fruit Crumble

2 portions stewed fruit, sweetened with fructose
3 oz (75g) soft margarine (milk-free if necessary)
4 oz (100g) ground rice
½ oz (15g) fructose

Put the fruit into an ovenproof dish and flatten the top. Weigh all other ingredients into a mixing bowl and rub in the margarine until the mixture resembles bread-crumbs. Sprinkle the mixture over the fruit, completely covering it. Make a hole in the middle right through to the fruit to let out the steam during cooking and bake at 425°F/220°C (Gas Mark 7) for about 10 minutes on the top shelf of the oven. Serve hot or cold. Makes 2–3 helpings.

Note: The fruit can be varied: dried apricots, prunes, mixed-fruit salad, dried peaches; fresh fruits in season – apricots, plums, gooseberries, blackcurrants, apple, blackberry and apple, apple and raspberry, pears, rhubarb etc.

• Suitable for all diets in this book.

Exotic Fruit Salad

1 orange, peeled and cut into slices
2 kiwi fruit, peeled and sliced thickly
1 banana, sliced
1 passion fruit, cut in half with seeds and pulp removed
¼ ripe melon, peeled and de-seeded, cut into cubes
handful of ripe, hulled strawberries, halved
fructose to taste

Combine prepared fruit in a bowl and sprinkle with fructose. Serve as soon as possible for maximum vitamin C value. If you prefer juice with the fruit salad squeeze over the juice of an orange.

• Suitable for all diets in this book.

Appendix

Further Reading

Manual of Nutrition. Published by the Ministry of Agriculture, Fisheries and Food and available from HM Stationery Office or bookshops.

Help Fight MS: Dietary Therapy with Polyunsaturated Fatty Acids by Dr Paul Evers, Klinik Dr Evers, 5768 Sundern-Langsheid, West Germany.

Multiple Sclerosis: A Self-Help Guide to its Management by Judy Graham (Thorsons).

Recommended Special Dietary Items and Where to Get Them*

Oil of Evening Primrose Capsules, *Cantamac, Foresight* Vitamins and Minerals, Vitamin B_{12} (1000mcg), Vitamin C (500 mcg), A, D and E, all made by Larkhall Green Farm who provide a mail order service (post free) from Department MSD, Larkhall Green Farm, 225 Putney Bridge Road, London SW15 2PY. Send s.a.e. for details. (Telephone: 0181-874-1130). This company also gives free advice/literature on gluten/wheat free diet.

Trufree flours (Nos. 1 to 7 100 per cent gluten-free and wheat-free) can be obtained by post from Larkhall Green Farm or from most branches of large chemists. (These may have to be ordered). Some smaller chemists also stock these items.

Fructose, Vitamins and *Minerals* are available from Health Food Stores.

Vitamins A and D are available as cod liver and halibut liver oil from most Chemists and Health Food Stores.

Buttermilk and skimmed milk is available from most supermarkets.

Tamari wheat/gluten-free soy sauce can be obtained from health stores.

Soya milk and milk free margarine are available from Health Food Stores and supermarkets.

* These are items which the author, in her experience, has found to be particularly suitable to her purpose. There are, though, alternatives on the market to a number of the items listed, but in all cases readers are advised to carefully read the labels before buying.

HEALING THROUGH NUTRITION

A NATURAL APPROACH TO TREATING 50 COMMON ILLNESSES WITH DIET AND NUTRIENTS

Dr Melvyn R. Werbach

This indispensable reference book provides the nutritional roots of and treatments for 50 common illnesses, from allergies and the common cold to cancer.

The world's authority on the relationship between nutrition and illness, Dr Melvyn Werbach makes it easy to learn what you can do to influence the course of your health via the nutrients that you feed your body.

A chapter is devoted to each of the 50 ailments and this highly accessible A–Z of nutritional health includes:

- an analysis of dietary factors affecting health and well-being
- a suggested healing diet for 50 common illnesses
- nutritional healing plans, with recommended dosages for vitamins, minerals and other essential nutrients
- an explanation of vitamin supplements and how they can improve your health

There are also guidelines on how to plan the right healing diet for yourself and how to diagnose food sensitivities. With this groundbreaking guide you will be able to make informed decisions about the essential role of nutrients in your health and well-being.

THE BOOK OF PAIN RELIEF	0 7225 2820 5	£7.99	☐
HEALING THROUGH NUTRITION	0 7225 2941 5	£16.99	☐
MULTIPLE SCLEROSIS	0 7225 2777 2	£9.99	☐
LET'S EAT RIGHT TO KEEP FIT	0 7225 3203 2	£5.99	☐

All these books are available from your local bookseller or can be ordered direct from the publishers.

To order direct just tick the titles you want and fill in the form below:

Name: _____

Address: _____

_____

_____ Postcode: _____

Send to: Thorsons Mail Order, Dept 3, HarperCollins*Publishers*, Westerhill Road, Bishopbriggs, Glasgow G64 2QT.
Please enclose a cheque or postal order or your authority to debit your Visa/Access account –

Credit card no: _____

Expiry date: _____

Signature: _____

– to the value of the cover price plus:
UK & BFPO: Add £1.00 for the first book and 25p for each additional book ordered.
Overseas orders including Eire: Please add £2.95 service charge. Books will be sent by surface mail but quotes for air-mail despatches will be given on request.

24 HOUR TELEPHONE ORDERING SERVICE FOR ACCESS/VISA CARDHOLDERS – **TEL: 0141 772 2281.**